AFFIRMATIONS FOR DIVINE HEALTH AND HEALING

THE MAKARIOS WAY

Walking in Health and Wellness Through Affirmation

MOSES FEEHI

Dedication

To God, the ultimate source of life, health, and healing—continue to walk in divine strength, embrace wholeness, and experience the power of His restoration in every area of your life. This book is dedicated to your journey toward divine health, inner peace, and the abundant healing promised to you.

CONTENTS

INTRODUCTION

Introduction to *Affirmations for Divine Health and Healing: The Makarios Way*

In our walk through life, health and well-being are fundamental pillars that directly influence our ability to live fully and fulfill our God-given purpose. For those who believe in divine health, affirmations grounded in faith and scripture become powerful tools to strengthen our connection to God's promises, promote healing, and live in wholeness.

The Importance of Divine Health Affirmations

Affirmations for divine health and healing are much more than mere positive statements; they are faith-filled declarations, aligning our hearts, minds, and bodies with the truth of God's Word. Here's why these affirmations are vital:

1. Reinforce Faith: Affirmations rooted in scripture serve as reminders of God's promises for healing and wholeness. Speaking them aloud renews our trust in His power to restore our health and keeps our faith strong, even in challenging times.

2. Shift Mindset: Regularly declaring affirmations helps redirect our focus from sickness and worry to God's promises. This mental shift can promote peace, reduce stress, and remind us that our ultimate healer is Christ, not just medical solutions.

3. Invoke God's Power: Affirmations activate our faith and invite God's divine power to work in our bodies. As we declare God's Word over our lives, we align our faith with His will for health and healing, allowing His supernatural power to manifest.

4. Promote Holistic Wellness: Repeated declarations based on God's Word contribute to overall health—spiritually, emotionally, and physically. As we affirm divine health, we tap into a higher level of wellness that encompasses body, soul, and spirit, enabling us to live as God intended.

These divine health affirmations will guide you to embrace God's promises, leading to a healthier, stronger, and more vibrant life through the power of faith.

HOW TO USE THIS BOOK

This affirmation book is designed to be a daily guide for embracing divine health and healing. Here's how to effectively use it:

1. Begin with Prayer and the Use the Name of Jesus: Start each session by praying in the name of Jesus. Acknowledge God as the source of all healing as you declare these affirmations.

2. Daily Practice: After prayer, read and speak a selection of affirmations aloud. Speaking in the name of Jesus adds power to your declarations, reinforcing your faith in God's healing promises.

3. Meditate on Scripture: Each affirmation is paired with a Bible verse. Take time to meditate on the Word of God, reflecting on how it applies to your health and healing. This deepens your faith and helps align your spirit with God's promises.

4. Personalize Your Affirmations: Adapt the affirmations to reflect your specific health needs or challenges. Incorporating the name of Jesus in these personalized statements increases the spiritual authority behind your words.

5. Speak with Belief: Declare each affirmation with confidence and belief, trusting in the power of Jesus' name to bring about healing and restoration. Remember, God's Word is powerful, and by speaking in faith, you activate that power in your life.

6. Combine with Prayer: Use the affirmations alongside your daily prayers. Continue to ask for God's intervention and healing, sealing your declarations in Jesus' name, knowing that the Lord hears and answers prayers made in faith.

7. Consistency is Key: Make this practice a consistent part of your routine. The more frequently you declare these truths in the name of Jesus, the stronger your faith will become and the deeper the affirmations will resonate in your life.

The Benefits of Using This Book

1. Strengthened Faith: Daily affirmations, especially when combined with prayer and the name of Jesus, reinforce your belief in God's healing power, giving you spiritual strength and confidence.

2. Increased Peace: Focusing on God's promises and praying in the name of Jesus helps reduce stress and anxiety, promoting a profound sense of peace and well-being.

3. Enhanced Healing: By declaring and believing in the name of Jesus, you invite His healing power into your life, potentially accelerating physical and emotional recovery.

4. Positive Mindset: Regular use of affirmations fosters hope and resilience, helping you maintain a positive outlook on your health and wellness journey.

5. Alignment with God's Will: Affirming your health in the name of Jesus aligns your thoughts and actions with God's divine will, ensuring that your path to wellness is blessed and guided by His Spirit.

Incorporating prayer, scripture, and the power of Jesus' name into your daily routine will bring about a transformative experience. Trust in God's promises, walk in faith, and declare His healing over your life with boldness and conviction.

AFFIRMATIONS 1

1. By His stripes, I am healed.

(Isaiah 53:5)

"But He was pierced for our transgressions, He was crushed for our iniquities; the punishment that brought us peace was on Him, and by His wounds we are healed."

2. I walk in divine health and wholeness, for my body is the temple of the Holy Spirit.

(1 Corinthians 6:19)

"Do you not know that your bodies are temples of the Holy Spirit, who is in you, whom you have received from God? You are not your own."

3. My health is restored and my wounds are healed.

(Jeremiah 30:17)

*"But I will restore you to health and heal your wounds,'
declares the Lord."*

4. I declare that no weapon formed against my health shall prosper.

(Isaiah 54:17)

*"No weapon forged against you will prevail, and you will
refute every tongue that accuses you. This is the heritage of
the servants of the Lord, and this is their vindication from
Me, declares the Lord."*

5. God renews my strength like the eagles; I run and do not grow weary.

(Isaiah 40:31)

"But those who hope in the Lord will renew their strength. They will soar on wings like eagles; they will run and not grow weary, they will walk and not be faint."

6. I speak life and healing over every part of my body.

(Proverbs 18:21)

"The tongue has the power of life and death, and those who love it will eat its fruit."

7. God has redeemed me from sickness and disease.

(Galatians 3:13)

"Christ redeemed us from the curse of the law by becoming a curse for us, for it is written: 'Cursed is everyone who is hung on a pole.'"

8. I am fearfully and wonderfully made, and every part of me functions as God designed.

(Psalm 139:14)

"I praise You because I am fearfully and wonderfully made; Your works are wonderful, I know that full well."

9. The Lord is my healer, and I trust in His healing power.

(Exodus 15:26)

"He said, 'If you listen carefully to the Lord your God and do what is right in His eyes, if you pay attention to His commands and keep all His decrees, I will not bring on you any of the diseases I brought on the Egyptians, for I am the Lord, who heals you.'"

10. I am strong, healthy, and vibrant, filled with God's life-giving power.

(John 10:10)

"The thief comes only to steal and kill and destroy; I have come that they may have life, and have it to the full."

A WORD FOR YOU 1

God's will for you is to walk in divine health and healing. The Bible is filled with promises of restoration and strength. When you face sickness or health challenges, it's essential to remember that healing is not just a future hope but a present reality made available through Jesus Christ.

God's Word is Healing: The Bible is clear that God's Word itself brings healing. Proverbs 4:20-22 says, *"My son, pay attention to what I say; turn your ear to My words. Do not let them out of your sight, keep them within your heart; for they are life to those who find them and health to one's whole body."* Meditating on God's Word regularly can bring supernatural healing to your body.

Faith is Key: In Mark 11:24, Jesus says, *"Therefore I tell you, whatever you ask for in prayer, believe that you have received it, and it will be yours."* Faith plays a crucial role in receiving healing. By affirming God's promises with belief, you allow His power to flow into your life.

Jesus' Healing Ministry: In His earthly ministry, Jesus healed countless people. Hebrews 13:8 tells us that *"Jesus Christ is the same yesterday and today and forever."* This means His desire to heal has not changed. The same power that healed the sick in the Bible is available to us today.

Healing is a Part of Redemption: When Jesus died on the cross, He not only carried our sins but also our sicknesses. Matthew 8:17 says, *"This was to fulfill what was spoken through the prophet Isaiah: 'He took up our infirmities and bore our diseases.'"* Because of this, healing is part of the salvation package for every believer.

Let these truths encourage you as you affirm divine health over your life. Trust that God is your healer, and that He is faithful to His Word. Healing is yours today through the power of Jesus Christ. Walk boldly in the strength and wellness He has provided, knowing that His promises are true.

AFFIRMATION 2

11. My immune system is strengthened by the power of God.

(Psalm 103:3)

"He forgives all your sins and heals all your diseases."
God is the source of all healing.

12. Every cell in my body responds to the life of Christ within me.

(Colossians 1:27)

"To them God has chosen to make known among the Gentiles the glorious riches of this mystery, which is Christ in you, the hope of glory."

13. I am healed from the crown of my head to the soles of my feet.

(Matthew 8:17)

"This was to fulfill what was spoken through the prophet Isaiah: 'He took up our infirmities and bore our diseases.'"

14. The joy of the Lord is my strength, and I receive His peace in my mind and body.

(Nehemiah 8:10)

"Nehemiah said, 'Go and enjoy choice food and sweet drinks, and send some to those who have nothing prepared. This day is holy to our Lord. Do not grieve, for the joy of the Lord is your strength.'"

15. I am not afraid of sickness, for God is with me and protects me.

(Psalm 91:10-11)

"No harm will overtake you, no disaster will come near your tent. For He will command His angels concerning you to guard you in all your ways."

16. I prosper and live in good health, just as my soul prospers.

(3 John 1:2)

"Dear friend, I pray that you may enjoy good health and that all may go well with you, even as your soul is getting along well."

17. God's Word is medicine to my body, bringing healing and restoration.

(Proverbs 4:20-22)

"My son, pay attention to what I say; turn your ear to My words. Do not let them out of your sight, keep them within your heart; for they are life to those who find them and health to one's whole body."

18. I release all fear and anxiety, knowing that God's perfect love heals me.

(1 John 4:18)

"There is no fear in love. But perfect love drives out fear, because fear has to do with punishment. The one who fears is not made perfect in love."

19. I stand in faith, knowing that healing is my portion as a child of God.
(Mark 5:34)

"He said to her, 'Daughter, your faith has healed you. Go in peace and be freed from your suffering.'"

20. I reject sickness, and I declare that health flows through me by the power of the Holy Spirit.
(Romans 8:11)

"And if the Spirit of Him who raised Jesus from the dead is living in you, He who raised Christ from the dead will also give life to your mortal bodies because of His Spirit who lives in you."

A WORD FOR YOU 2

God desires that you walk in divine health, and His Word is filled with promises that affirm His power and willingness to heal. As you meditate on these scriptures and speak these affirmations over your life, remember that healing is not only a gift for the future, but it is available to you now, through faith in Jesus Christ.

The Healing Power of God's Word: As declared in Proverbs 4:20-22, God's Word is medicine to our bodies. Regularly meditating on and declaring His promises activates the healing power of the Word. Make it a daily practice to feed on scripture as you would a necessary nutrient for your physical health.

Faith Moves Mountains: Jesus repeatedly acknowledged the role of faith in healing. In Mark 11:24, He said, *"Therefore I tell you, whatever you ask for in prayer, believe that you have received it, and it will be yours."* Faith is the key that unlocks the door to divine healing. Believe that God is able and willing to heal, and expect His touch in your life.

Jesus, Our Healer: The ministry of Jesus was filled with healing miracles, showing us that healing is God's will for His children. Hebrews 13:8 reminds us that *"Jesus Christ is the same yesterday and today and forever."* The same healing power that was at work during Jesus' time on earth is available to you today.

Divine Healing as Part of Redemption: Healing is not just a blessing for a select few—it is part of the redemption Jesus purchased on the cross. In Isaiah 53:5, we read that *"by His stripes, we are healed."* When Jesus bore our sins, He also bore our sicknesses. As believers, we have the right to claim this healing.

As you declare these affirmations and meditate on the scriptures, let your faith grow stronger. Healing is not just a wish—it is a promise. Stand on God's Word, trust in His love, and walk confidently in the divine health He has provided for you through Jesus Christ.

21. I am healed and made whole by the power of Jesus' name.

(Acts 3:16)

"By faith in the name of Jesus, this man whom you see and know was made strong. It is Jesus' name and the faith that comes through Him that has completely healed him, as you can all see."

22. Every disease, every ailment is defeated by the blood of Jesus.

(Revelation 12:11)

"They triumphed over him by the blood of the Lamb and by the word of their testimony; they did not love their lives so much as to shrink from death."

23. God's healing power is active in my life, restoring me to perfect health.

(Psalm 107:20)

"He sent out His word and healed them; He rescued them from the grave."

24. I walk in the light of God's healing grace, and I am free from sickness.

(1 John 1:7)

"But if we walk in the light, as He is in the light, we have fellowship with one another, and the blood of Jesus, His Son, purifies us from all sin."

25. The Lord's healing virtue flows through me, bringing restoration and vitality.

(Luke 6:19)

"And the people all tried to touch Him, because power was coming from Him and healing them all."

26. I trust in God's promises of health and healing, knowing He is faithful.

(2 Peter 3:9)

"The Lord is not slow in keeping His promise, as some understand slowness. Instead, He is patient with you, not wanting anyone to perish, but everyone to come to repentance."

27. I am covered by God's protection and healing power.

(Psalm 91:4)

"He will cover you with His feathers, and under His wings you will find refuge; His faithfulness will be your shield and rampart."

28. I am made new and whole by the power of Christ's resurrection.

(Romans 8:11)

"And if the Spirit of Him who raised Jesus from the dead is living in you, He who raised Christ from the dead will also give life to your mortal bodies because of His Spirit who lives in you."

29. God has given me a spirit of power, love, and a sound mind.

(2 Timothy 1:7)

"For the Spirit God gave us does not make us timid, but gives us power, love, and self-discipline."

30. I declare that my body is strong and healed, for God is my healer.

(Exodus 23:25)

"Worship the Lord your God, and His blessing will be on your food and water. I will take away sickness from among you."

A WORD FOR YOU 3

The power of God's Word is alive and active, bringing healing and wholeness to every area of our lives. As you meditate on these affirmations and scriptures, be encouraged that divine health is your portion as a child of God.

The Power of Jesus' Name: In Acts 3:16, we see the incredible power of the name of Jesus to heal. The same power is available to you today. When you call on Jesus' name, believe that healing will manifest, just as it did for those who encountered Him in the Gospels.

Victory through the Blood of Jesus: The blood of Jesus has triumphed over every sickness. Revelation 12:11 reminds us that by His blood, we have overcome. This victory is yours to claim—speak it over your body and every circumstance you face.

God's Word Heals: As Psalm 107:20 declares, God sends His Word to heal and deliver. His Word is not passive but active, working to restore you to full health. Declare these scriptures daily, knowing that they are accomplishing God's purpose in your life.

Resurrection Power at Work: Romans 8:11 promises that the same Spirit who raised Jesus from the dead gives life to your mortal body. This life-giving power is working in you right now, bringing healing, strength, and vitality. Never doubt the transformative power of God's Spirit within you.

Standing in Faith: Like the woman with the issue of blood in Mark 5:34, your faith can make you whole. Stand firm in your faith, knowing that healing is not just possible but promised to you by your Heavenly Father. Believe that as you declare these affirmations, healing is taking place in your body, mind, and spirit.

God's will for you is complete health—body, soul, and spirit. As you continue to meditate on these affirmations, trust in His promises and allow His healing power to flow freely through your life. Stay rooted in His Word, speak it with faith, and watch as His healing touch brings you into perfect wholeness.

AFFIRMATIONS 4

31. The Lord heals me and makes me whole, bringing peace to my body and mind.

(Psalm 147:3)

"He heals the brokenhearted and binds up their wounds."

32. I am redeemed from every sickness and disease by the blood of Jesus.

(1 Peter 2:24)

"He Himself bore our sins in His body on the cross, so that we might die to sins and live for righteousness; by His wounds you have been healed."

33. My body is energized and revitalized by the power of God.

(Isaiah 40:29)

"He gives strength to the weary and increases the power of the weak."

34. I am filled with God's life and health, and I experience His divine healing.

(John 6:63)

"The Spirit gives life; the flesh counts for nothing. The words I have spoken to you—they are full of the Spirit and life."

35. God's healing presence surrounds me, bringing comfort and recovery.

(Psalm 34:18)

"The Lord is close to the brokenhearted and saves those who are crushed in spirit."

36. I am free from all forms of illness and live in divine health through Christ.

(Matthew 10:8)

"Heal the sick, raise the dead, cleanse those who have leprosy, drive out demons. Freely you have received; freely give."

37. The Lord's healing power is at work within me, restoring me to full health.

(Philippians 2:13)

"For it is God who works in you to will and to act in order to fulfill His good purpose."

38. I reject every lie of sickness and embrace God's truth of healing.

(John 8:32)

"Then you will know the truth, and the truth will set you free."

39. I am strengthened by God's grace and empowered for health and vitality.

(2 Corinthians 12:9)

"But He said to me, 'My grace is sufficient for you, for my power is made perfect in weakness.'"

40. God's healing Word is effective in my life, bringing wholeness to every part of me.

(Isaiah 55:11)

"So is My word that goes out from My mouth: It will not return to Me empty, but will accomplish what I desire and achieve the purpose for which I sent it."

A WORD FOR YOU 4

God's Word is powerful, living, and active, and it brings life to all who believe in it. The promises of healing are written throughout scripture, reaffirming that divine health is a gift from God for His children. As you meditate on these affirmations and scriptures, remember these truths:

The Power of the Blood of Jesus: According to 1 Peter 2:24, the sacrifice of Jesus ensures that healing is already accomplished. By His wounds, you have been healed. Declare this over your body and believe that every sickness is defeated by the power of His blood.

God's Healing Presence: Psalm 34:18 reminds us that God is near to those who need comfort and healing. His presence brings supernatural restoration, guiding you through every step of recovery and wellness. Trust that His nearness is bringing peace and health to you.

Strength in Weakness: As 2 Corinthians 12:9 assures, God's grace is sufficient for you. In times of physical or emotional weakness, rely on His power. His strength is made perfect in your moments of need, ensuring that His grace carries you into full health and vitality.

Healing is God's Will: Isaiah 55:11 tells us that God's Word never returns void. His promises of healing will be fulfilled in your life as you declare them in faith. Trust that His Word is working within you, bringing complete restoration to your body, mind, and spirit.

In moments of doubt or sickness, remember that God's will is for you to walk in divine health. These affirmations and scriptures are not just words—they are spiritual weapons that activate God's healing power in your life. Stay rooted in His Word, speak His promises daily, and believe that healing is already yours.

AFFIRMATIONS 5

41. I am healed from all afflictions because of God's unchanging love.

(Psalm 103:2-3)

"Praise the Lord, my soul, and forget not all His benefits—who forgives all your sins and heals all your diseases."

42. God's power is made perfect in my weakness, and His strength sustains me.

(2 Corinthians 12:9)

"But He said to me, 'My grace is sufficient for you, for my power is made perfect in weakness.'"

43. I embrace God's promise of health and reject the spirit of infirmity.

(Luke 13:11-12)

"When Jesus saw her, He called her forward and said to her, 'Woman, you are set free from your infirmity.'"

44. The healing power of God restores every organ and system in my body.

(Jeremiah 33:6)

"Nevertheless, I will bring health and healing to it; I will heal My people and will let them enjoy abundant peace and security."

45. I am covered by God's healing protection, and no evil shall come near me.

(Psalm 91:10)

"No harm will overtake you, no disaster will come near your tent."

46. God's divine health flows through me, bringing strength and vitality to my body.

(1 Peter 2:24)

"He Himself bore our sins in His body on the cross, so that we might die to sins and live for righteousness; by His wounds you have been healed."

47. I claim God's healing promises over my life and experience His supernatural health.

(Mark 16:18)

"...they will place their hands on sick people, and they will get well."

48. Every symptom of illness is cast out, and I walk in the fullness of God's healing.

(Matthew 17:20)

"He replied, 'Because you have so little faith. Truly I tell you, if you have faith as small as a mustard seed, you can say to this mountain, "Move from here to there," and it will move. Nothing will be impossible for you.'"

49. I am rejuvenated by the power of God's Spirit, and my health is restored.

(Romans 8:11)

"And if the Spirit of Him who raised Jesus from the dead is living in you, He who raised Christ from the dead will also give life to your mortal bodies because of His Spirit who lives in you."

50. The Lord is my healer; I trust in His power to deliver me from all sickness.

(Exodus 15:26)

"He said, 'If you listen carefully to the Lord your God and do what is right in His eyes, if you pay attention to His commands and keep all His decrees, I will not bring on you any of the diseases I brought on the Egyptians, for I am the Lord, who heals you.'"

A WORD OF YOU 5

Healing is an integral part of God's plan for His children. As believers, you have been given access to divine health and healing through Christ. When you declare these affirmations, you are not only speaking positive words but also aligning yourself with God's promises in Scripture. Here are some important truths to hold onto:

Healing is a Gift: As mentioned in 1 Peter 2:24, by the stripes of Jesus, you are healed. Healing is not something you have to earn; it is a gift from God, already paid for by the sacrifice of Jesus Christ. Stand firm in the knowledge that healing is your inheritance as a child of God.

The Power of God's Word: God's Word is living and active, sharper than any double-edged sword (Hebrews 4:12). The scriptures you declare have the power to bring healing and restoration. As Isaiah 55:11 assures, God's Word will not return void but will accomplish what it was sent to do. As you speak His promises, healing is released into your life.

Faith is Key: Throughout the Gospels, Jesus emphasizes faith as a key to receiving healing. In Mark 5:34, Jesus tells the woman with the issue of blood, "Your faith has healed you." Continue to nurture your faith through prayer, meditation on the Word, and daily affirmations. Faith, even as small as a mustard seed, can move mountains, including the mountain of sickness (Matthew 17:20).

God's Will is Healing: Exodus 15:26 reveals God's heart toward healing: "I am the Lord, who heals you." His will is not for you to suffer in sickness but to experience wholeness and vitality. Trust that His will for you is divine health, and by aligning your thoughts and declarations with His Word, you are opening yourself to His healing touch.

Stay steadfast in faith, continue to declare these affirmations, and trust that God's healing power is at work in your life. Healing belongs to you in Christ, and as you stand on these truths, you will experience the fullness of health and vitality that God desires for you.

AFFIRMATIONS 6

51. I am completely healed, and my body functions as God intended.
(Colossians 1:16-17)

"For in Him all things were created: things in heaven and on earth, visible and invisible... all things have been created through Him and for Him. He is before all things, and in Him, all things hold together."

52. God's healing touch removes all pain and restores my strength.
(Luke 4:40)

"At sunset, the people brought to Jesus all who had various kinds of sickness, and laying His hands on each one, He healed them."

53. I declare divine health and reject any form of disease or disorder.

(Proverbs 4:20-22)

"My son, pay attention to what I say; turn your ear to my words. Do not let them out of your sight, keep them within your heart; for they are life to those who find them and health to one's whole body."

54. The Lord gives me strength and vitality; I am made whole in Him.

(Isaiah 12:2)

"Surely God is my salvation; I will trust and not be afraid. The Lord, the Lord Himself, is my strength and my defense; He has become my salvation."

55. I am healed from the inside out by the power of God's Word.

(Hebrews 4:12)

"For the word of God is alive and active. Sharper than any double-edged sword, it penetrates even to dividing soul and spirit, joints and marrow; it judges the thoughts and attitudes of the heart."

56. God's promises of healing and health are alive and active in my life.

(2 Corinthians 1:20)

"For no matter how many promises God has made, they are 'Yes' in Christ. And so through Him, the 'Amen' is spoken by us to the glory of God."

57. I experience divine health and live in the fullness of God's healing power.

(Deuteronomy 7:15)

"The Lord will keep you free from every disease. He will not inflict on you the horrible diseases you knew in Egypt, but He will inflict them on all who hate you."

58. I am anointed for health and wholeness, and every part of me is renewed.

(Acts 10:38)

"...how God anointed Jesus of Nazareth with the Holy Spirit and power, and how He went around doing good and healing all who were under the power of the devil, because God was with Him."

59. God's healing grace covers every area of my life, bringing peace and recovery.

(2 Corinthians 12:9)

"But He said to me, 'My grace is sufficient for you, for my power is made perfect in weakness.' Therefore I will boast all the more gladly about my weaknesses, so that Christ's power may rest on me."

60. I stand firm in faith, knowing that God's healing is working in me.

(James 5:15)

"And the prayer offered in faith will make the sick person well; the Lord will raise them up."

A WORD FOR YOU 6

God's desire is for you to live in divine health and experience the fullness of His healing power. As you continue to speak these affirmations over your life, you are aligning yourself with the truth of His Word, which is living and active (Hebrews 4:12), and bringing health to your whole body (Proverbs 4:22). The Bible repeatedly assures us that healing is part of the salvation package Christ purchased for us on the cross:

Healing Through Faith: Faith is the key to accessing divine healing. Jesus repeatedly told those He healed, "Your faith has made you well" (Mark 5:34). When you declare these affirmations in faith, you are positioning yourself to receive God's healing touch.

The Power of God's Word: As you speak God's Word, it works within you, bringing life to your bones and health to your body. Proverbs 18:21 reminds us that life and death are in the power of the tongue. Speak life by declaring God's promises, and watch as His Word accomplishes what it was sent to do (Isaiah 55:11).

God's Will is Health: Throughout Scripture, God shows His desire for His people to walk in health. Exodus 15:26 says, "I am the Lord who heals you." It is not His will for you to be sick, but to be whole. Trust in His desire to heal you as you stand on His promises.

Christ's Sacrifice Brings Healing: 1 Peter 2:24 affirms that by Christ's wounds, we are healed. This healing is not just spiritual but encompasses every area of your life. Through Christ's sacrifice, healing has been made available to you.

Remain steadfast in your faith, declare these truths with confidence, and trust that God's healing power is active in your life. Healing is yours through Christ, and as you walk in His promises, you will experience divine health and wholeness.

AFFIRMATIONS 7

61. The healing power of Christ is at work in my body, bringing restoration and health.

(Matthew 8:3)

"Jesus reached out His hand and touched the man. 'I am willing,' He said. 'Be clean!' Immediately he was cleansed of his leprosy."

62. I am blessed with divine health, and my body is free from disease.

(Proverbs 3:8)

"This will bring health to your body and nourishment to your bones."

63. I receive God's healing power and walk in divine health every day.

(Isaiah 53:5)

"But He was pierced for our transgressions, He was crushed for our iniquities; the punishment that brought us peace was on Him, and by His wounds, we are healed."

64. God's love for me ensures my complete healing and restoration.

(Romans 8:37)

"No, in all these things we are more than conquerors through Him who loved us."

65. I am strengthened by God's might and healed by His power.

(Ephesians 6:10)

"Finally, be strong in the Lord and in His mighty power."

66. I declare that sickness has no place in my body; I am healed in Jesus' name.

(John 14:14)

"You may ask me for anything in my name, and I will do it."

67. The Lord is my healer, and I walk in His divine health and protection.

(Psalm 30:2)

"Lord my God, I called to You for help, and You healed me."

68. I am empowered by God's grace to experience perfect health and healing.

(2 Corinthians 12:9)

"But He said to me, 'My grace is sufficient for you, for My power is made perfect in weakness.'"

69. Every ailment and pain is healed by the power of Jesus' sacrifice.

(1 Peter 2:24)

"He Himself bore our sins in His body on the cross, so that we might die to sins and live for righteousness; by His wounds, you have been healed."

70. I am a recipient of God's abundant health and healing.

(John 10:10)

"The thief comes only to steal and kill and destroy; I have come that they may have life, and have it to the full."

A WORD FOR YOU 7

God's will for you is to walk in divine health and experience His healing power in every area of your life. Through the Word of God, you can stand firm in His promises of healing and restoration. Let these scriptures inspire you to deepen your faith and confidently receive His gift of health:

Healing is God's Will: In Psalm 103:2-3, David says, "Praise the Lord, my soul, and forget not all His benefits—who forgives all your sins and heals all your diseases." It is clear from Scripture that healing is one of the benefits God provides to His children. Believe that His will for you is to be healed and whole.

Faith Activates Healing: Hebrews 11:1 teaches that "faith is the substance of things hoped for, the evidence of things not seen." When you declare affirmations of healing, you are expressing faith in what you may not yet see. This faith is the key to accessing God's power and bringing healing into your life.

The Power of Christ's Sacrifice: Jesus took all your infirmities on Himself when He went to the cross. Isaiah 53:5 tells us that "by His wounds, we are healed." Christ has already paid the price for your health, and now it's up to you to receive and walk in the healing that He has freely given.

God's Word Brings Life: Proverbs 4:20-22 says, "My son, pay attention to what I say... for they are life to those who find them and health to one's whole body." The Word of God is alive and powerful, bringing life and health to your entire being. Meditate on His Word and let it saturate your heart and mind, bringing healing to your body.

Divine Protection and Health: Psalm 91:10-11 assures you of God's protection, saying, "no harm will overtake you, no disaster will come near your tent. For He will command His angels concerning you to guard you in all your ways." God promises to keep you safe and healthy, protected from sickness and disease.

In moments of sickness, it is essential to remember that God has already provided a way for you to be healed through Jesus Christ. Keep standing in faith, declaring these scriptures over your life, and trust that His healing power is working in you. Healing is your portion as a child of God, and as you continue to speak these truths, you will experience the fullness of health and wholeness that God desires for you.

71. God's healing virtue continually flows through my entire being.

(Luke 8:46)

"But Jesus said, 'Someone touched me; I know that power has gone out from me.'"

72. I am free from all sickness and live in the divine health provided by God.

(Psalm 91:3)

"Surely He will save you from the fowler's snare and from the deadly pestilence."

73. My health is restored and revitalized by the power of God's Word.

(Psalm 107:20)

"He sent out His word and healed them; He rescued them from the grave."

74. God's promise of healing is manifest in my life, bringing wholeness and vitality.

(Jeremiah 33:6)

"'Nevertheless, I will bring health and healing to it; I will heal My people and will let them enjoy abundant peace and security.'"

75. I am healed and made whole, experiencing God's complete restoration.

(1 Thessalonians 5:23)

"May God Himself, the God of peace, sanctify you through and through. May your whole spirit, soul, and body be kept blameless at the coming of our Lord Jesus Christ."

76. The power of God's healing is active in my life, bringing me renewed strength.

(Isaiah 40:29)

"He gives strength to the weary and increases the power of the weak."

77. I am blessed with good health and vitality, for the Lord is my healer.

(Exodus 23:25)

"Worship the Lord your God, and His blessing will be on your food and water. I will take away sickness from among you."

78. Every cell in my body responds to the healing power of God.

(Colossians 1:16)

"For in Him all things were created: things in heaven and on earth, visible and invisible, whether thrones or powers or rulers or authorities; all things have been created through Him and for Him."

79. I walk in divine health, protected and strengthened by the Lord.

(Psalm 91:10)

"No harm will overtake you, no disaster will come near your tent."

80. God's Word is a lamp to my feet and healing to my body.

(Proverbs 4:22)

"For they are life to those who find them and health to one's whole body."

A WORD FOR YOU 8

God's Word is filled with promises that ensure health and healing for His children. His desire for you is to live a life of vitality, free from the burden of sickness. As you meditate on the following scriptures, let them inspire your faith and remind you of God's unwavering commitment to your healing:

God's Will to Heal: Jeremiah 30:17 says, "But I will restore you to health and heal your wounds," declares the Lord. God's will is to restore you fully—to heal you and bring you to complete health. Trust in His intention and believe that healing is already yours.

Faith and Healing: Mark 11:24 teaches, "Therefore I tell you, whatever you ask for in prayer, believe that you have received it, and it will be yours." When you ask for healing, believe it is done, and through your faith, you will experience the fullness of God's promise of health.

Healing in His Name: In the name of Jesus, there is power to heal. John 14:13 assures us, "And I will do whatever you ask in My name, so that the Father may be glorified in the Son." As you speak in the name of Jesus, sickness is defeated, and His healing power is released into your life.

The Power of God's Word: Proverbs 4:20-22 speaks of the life-giving and healing power of God's Word: "My son, pay attention to what I say; turn your ear to My words. Do not let them out of your sight, keep them within your heart; for they are life to those who find them and health to one's whole body." His Word is alive and active, bringing healing to every part of your body.

Healing Through Jesus' Sacrifice: 1 Peter 2:24 reminds us that "by His wounds, you have been healed." Jesus took every sickness upon Himself at the cross, and because of His sacrifice, healing is now your inheritance. Declare this truth over your life, knowing that your healing has already been secured by Christ.

Keep holding on to these promises, and continue to declare them over your health. Healing is a covenant promise, and as you stand in faith, you will see the manifestation of God's complete restoration in your life. You are healed, whole, and walking in divine health as a beloved child of God.

AFFIRMATIONS 9

81. I reject every symptom of illness and embrace God's promise of perfect health.

(2 Timothy 1:7)

"For the Spirit God gave us does not make us timid, but gives us power, love, and self-discipline."

82. The Lord's healing grace restores me to full health and strength.

(Psalm 103:5)

"Who satisfies your desires with good things so that your youth is renewed like the eagle's."

83. I am covered by the healing power of Christ, and every disease is removed.

(Acts 5:16)

"Crowds gathered also from the towns around Jerusalem, bringing their sick and those tormented by impure spirits, and all of them were healed."

84. God's healing presence is evident in my life, bringing comfort and recovery.

(Psalm 147:3)

"He heals the brokenhearted and binds up their wounds."

85. I am rejuvenated and restored, walking in the fullness of God's healing.

(Isaiah 58:8)

"Then your light will break forth like the dawn, and your healing will quickly appear; then your righteousness will go before you, and the glory of the Lord will be your rear guard."

86. The Lord's healing power is at work in me, making me whole and healthy.

(Matthew 9:22)

"Jesus turned and saw her. 'Take heart, daughter,' He said, 'your faith has healed you.' And the woman was healed at that moment."

87. I am continually healed and renewed by the power of God's Spirit.

(Romans 8:11)

"And if the Spirit of Him who raised Jesus from the dead is living in you, He who raised Christ from the dead will also give life to your mortal bodies because of His Spirit who lives in you."

88. I claim divine health and reject any form of sickness or disease.

(Mark 16:18)

"They will place their hands on sick people, and they will get well."

89. God's promise of healing is fulfilled in my life, bringing peace and restoration.

(2 Corinthians 1:20)

"For no matter how many promises God has made, they are 'Yes' in Christ. And so through Him, the 'Amen' is spoken by us to the glory of God."

90. I am strengthened and invigorated by the healing power of Jesus.

(John 11:4)

"When He heard this, Jesus said, 'This sickness will not end in death. No, it is for God's glory so that God's Son may be glorified through it.'"

A WORD FOR YOU

The healing promises of God are a powerful reminder of His love and care for us. God's desire is for you to walk in complete health, free from the grip of sickness. Here are key scriptures to inspire your faith as you continue to stand on God's promises of healing:

God is Your Healer: In Exodus 15:26, God declares, "I am the Lord who heals you." He is your ultimate Healer, and His healing power is always available to you. Trust in His love and His ability to restore you to perfect health.

Faith Brings Healing: Mark 5:34 reminds us, "Daughter, your faith has healed you. Go in peace and be freed from your suffering." Like the woman with the issue of blood, your faith activates healing. Trust God's power and believe that He is working in your body right now.

Power in the Name of Jesus: John 14:14 says, "You may ask me for anything in my name, and I will do it." Healing is yours in the name of Jesus. Speak His name over your life, knowing that there is power in His name to heal and restore every part of your being.

God's Word Brings Life and Health: Proverbs 4:22 speaks of the healing power of God's Word: "For they are life to those who find them and health to one's whole body." God's Word is like medicine to your soul, bringing health and life to every part of your body. As you meditate on His Word, healing flows through you.

By His Wounds, You Are Healed: 1 Peter 2:24 states, "By His wounds you have been healed." Jesus took your sickness upon Himself at the cross. His suffering secured your healing. Declare this truth over your life, knowing that healing is your inheritance because of what Jesus accomplished.

As you hold fast to these scriptures, believe that God is working in your life, healing you from every sickness, pain, and ailment. Keep speaking His promises, stand firm in your faith, and you will experience the fullness of His healing power. You are healed, restored, and walking in divine health as a child of God!

AFFIRMATIONS 10

91. The Lord restores my health and delivers me from all afflictions.

(Psalm 41:3)

"The Lord sustains them on their sickbed and restores them from their bed of illness."

92. I walk in God's divine health, protected and healed from every infirmity.

(Psalm 91:16)

"With long life I will satisfy him and show him my salvation."

93. I am revitalized by the power of God's Word, and my health is restored.

(Isaiah 55:11)

"So is my word that goes out from my mouth: It will not return to me empty, but will accomplish what I desire and achieve the purpose for which I sent it."

94. God's healing grace surrounds me, bringing recovery and vitality.

(Isaiah 53:5)

"But He was pierced for our transgressions, He was crushed for our iniquities; the punishment that brought us peace was on Him, and by His wounds we are healed."

95. I declare that I am healed and live in the fullness of God's health.

(James 5:14)

"Is anyone among you sick? Let them call the elders of the church to pray over them and anoint them with oil in the name of the Lord."

96. The power of God's healing is evident in my life, making me whole and strong.

(Psalm 103:2-3)

"Praise the Lord, my soul, and forget not all His benefits— who forgives all your sins and heals all your diseases."

97. I am healed and restored by the power of God's Word, which brings life to my body.

(Proverbs 4:22)

"For they are life to those who find them and health to one's whole body."

98. God's healing touch is evident in my life, bringing health and wholeness.

(Luke 8:50)

"Hearing this, Jesus said to Jairus, 'Don't be afraid; just believe, and she will be healed.'"

99. I walk in the promise of divine health, knowing that God is my healer.

(Exodus 15:26)

"He said, 'If you listen carefully to the Lord your God and do what is right in His eyes, if you pay attention to His commands and keep all His decrees, I will not bring on you any of the diseases I brought on the Egyptians, for I am the Lord, who heals you.'"

100. I am empowered by God's strength and live in divine health, free from all disease.

(Psalm 29:11)

"The Lord gives strength to His people; the Lord blesses His people with peace."

A WORD FOR YOU 10

God's desire is for you to live in divine health, and His Word is filled with promises of healing and restoration. Here are some key scriptures to meditate on as you stand on God's Word for your health:

The Lord Is Your Healer: Exodus 15:26 declares, "I am the Lord, who heals you." Trust in God's identity as your healer. He is committed to restoring you and keeping you in divine health.

God's Word Brings Healing: Proverbs 4:20-22 reminds us, "My son, pay attention to what I say; turn your ear to my words. Do not let them out of your sight, keep them within your heart; for they are life to those who find them and health to one's whole body." As you meditate on His Word, it brings life and healing to every part of you.

Jesus Paid the Price for Your Healing: Isaiah 53:5 proclaims, "By His wounds, we are healed." Jesus took your sickness and disease on Himself at the cross. His sacrifice has already secured your healing—believe it and receive it today!

Healing Comes Through Faith: In Mark 5:34, Jesus says, "Daughter, your faith has healed you. Go in peace and be freed from your suffering." Like the woman who touched Jesus' garment, your faith can activate the healing power of God. Believe and receive your healing by faith.

The Power of Prayer for Healing: James 5:14-15 encourages, "Is anyone among you sick? Let them call the elders of the church to pray over them and anoint them with oil in the name of the Lord. And the prayer offered in faith will make the sick person well." The power of prayer and faith releases healing into your body. Seek prayer and stand in faith, knowing that God is faithful to heal.

As you declare these scriptures over your life, you are reminding yourself of God's unchanging promises. Let His Word fill your heart and mind, for it is the key to experiencing divine health and wholeness. You are healed, restored, and strengthened by the power of God's love and grace. Keep your faith strong, and walk in the fullness of His healing power every day!

CONCLUSION

As you come to the end of this journey of affirmations, prayers, and declarations, remember that God's Word is alive and powerful. Every truth, every scripture, and every affirmation you have declared over your life has the power to bring healing, restoration, and transformation. The Bible says that "death and life are in the power of the tongue" (Proverbs 18:21), and as you continue to speak life over your body, mind, and spirit, you are partnering with God's will for your health and wholeness.

The journey to health and healing is not always instant, but God is faithful. His Word never returns void but accomplishes what He has sent it to do (Isaiah 55:11). By standing on His promises, you are aligning yourself with His perfect will for your life. Continue to meditate on these scriptures and speak them over yourself daily, knowing that God is at work within you, bringing healing to every area of your life.

Your faith has the power to unlock the supernatural, and with every declaration, you are planting seeds of healing that will yield a harvest of health, strength, and vitality. Keep believing, keep speaking, and keep trusting in the God who heals.

A Word of Encouragement

Beloved, know that God loves you deeply and desires for you to walk in divine health. Whatever challenges you may be facing right now—whether physical, emotional, or spiritual—God is greater than any illness or infirmity. He is the Great Physician, the One who formed you in your mother's womb, and He knows every detail of your life.

Jesus paid the ultimate price for your healing on the cross. By His wounds, you are healed (Isaiah 53:5). As you stand on this truth, trust that God is working all things together for your good (Romans 8:28). No matter how long the process may seem, don't lose hope. Healing is not only God's will for you, but it is your inheritance as a child of God.

In moments of doubt or weariness, turn to Him in prayer. Call upon the name of Jesus, for His name is above every sickness, every disease, and every obstacle you face.

Remember, God's strength is made perfect in your weakness (2 Corinthians 12:9). When you feel weak, He is strong in you, carrying you through to victory.

You are not alone in this journey. God is with you, and His Spirit dwells within you, giving you life and strength (Romans 8:11). Continue to walk in faith, knowing that God's promises are sure. Healing is your portion, and His grace is sufficient for you.

May you always rest in the peace that surpasses all understanding, knowing that your God is faithful and that your healing is already secured through Jesus Christ. Keep pressing forward, for the Lord is your healer, your refuge, and your strength. You are healed, you are whole, and you are loved beyond measure. Keep believing and declaring His word, for your breakthrough is already on its way. Amen.

Prayer of Salvation

85

O Lord God, I come to you in the name of Jesus. Your word says whosoever shall call upon your name shall be saved. I believe in with all my heart that Jesus is the Son of the Living God. I declare with my mouth that Jesus is the Lord of my life from this day. I declare that I am saved. I am a child of God. Amen

IMPORTANT MATERIALS

The Bible: A timeless source of wisdom, guidance, and inspiration.

Affirmations for Children: The Makarios Way by Moses Feehi

A wonderful collection of affirmations aimed at helping children develop a strong sense of self-worth, faith, and resilience, all grounded in biblical principles.

Affirmations and Meditation for Students: The Makarios Way by Moses Feehi

A guide designed to empower students through affirmations and meditation, helping them build a strong foundation of faith, focus, and success.

Affirmations and Meditation for Business People: The Makarios Way by Moses Feehi

A powerful resource for business professionals, providing affirmations and meditations to inspire success, perseverance, and ethical leadership.

Affirmations for Men: The Makarios Way by Moses Feehi

A resource tailored to empower men with affirmations that promote strength, leadership, faith, and personal growth.

Affirmations for Women: The Makarios Way by Moses Feehi

A guide specifically for women, offering affirmations that encourage confidence, grace, faith, and empowerment in every aspect of life.

How to Handle Personal Finances: The Makarios Way by Moses Feehi

This practical guide offers essential strategies for managing your finances wisely. Learn how to budget, save, and invest effectively while aligning your financial decisions with your personal values.

Tracking Your Finances: The Makarios Way by Moses Feehi

This resource provides tools and techniques for monitoring your financial health. Discover methods to track expenses, set financial goals, and maintain accountability, ensuring you stay on the path to financial success.

The Power of Your Mind by Pastor Chris Oyakhilome
This insightful book explores the incredible capabilities of your mind and how harnessing its power can lead to personal transformation and success

Rhapsody of Realities Daily Devotional by Pastor Chris Oyakhilome: A wonderful tool to help young minds grow in faith, learn biblical principles, and apply them to everyday life.

Recreating Your World by Pastor Chris Oyakhilome
In this powerful work, Pastor Oyakhilome emphasizes the importance of aligning your thoughts with God's will to transform your life. Discover how to reshape your reality through faith, vision, and purpose